Copyright © 2020

All rights reserved. No part of this publication may be reproduced, distributed, or transmitted in any form or by any means, including photocopying, recording, or other electronic or mechanical methods, without the prior written permission of the publisher, except in the case of brief quotations embodied in critical reviews and certain other noncommercial uses permitted by copyright law.

Contents

Everything You Need to Know About Hypothyroidism ...7

What is hypothyroidism? ...7

What causes hypothyroidism? ...11

An autoimmune disease ...11

Treatment for hyperthyroidism ...12

Radiation therapy ...13

Medications ...14

Diagnosing hypothyroidism ...14

Medical evaluation ...15

Blood tests ...16

Medications for hypothyroidism ...17

Alternative treatment for hypothyroidism ...19

Eat a balanced diet ...21

Monitor soy intake 21

Be smart with fiber 22

Living with hypothyroidism: Things to consider 23

Develop fatigue coping strategies 23

Talk it out 24

Monitor for other health conditions 25

Hypothyroidism and depression 26

Hypothyroidism and anxiety 28

Hypothyroidism and pregnancy 29

Stay current on medicine 31

Talk to your doctor about testing 31

Eat well 32

Hypothyroidism and weight loss 32

Hypothyroidism and weight gain 34

Facts and statistics about hypothyroidism 35

10 Signs and Symptoms of Hypothyroidism 38

1. Feeling Tired 40

2. Gaining Weight 42

3. Feeling Cold 44

4. Weakness and Aches in Muscles and Joints 46

5. Hair Loss 48

6. Itchy and Dry Skin 50

7. Feeling Down or Depressed 52

8. Trouble Concentrating or Remembering 54

9. Constipation 55

10. Heavy or Irregular Periods 57

Your Hypothyroidism Diet Plan: Eat This, Not That 61

What to eat 61

What to limit or avoid 62

Iodine 63

Soy 64

Fiber 65

Cruciferous vegetables 65

Alcohol 66

Gluten 67

Iron and calcium 67

Planning your diet 68

Your Treatment Options for Hypothyroidism 69

Medications and Supplements 70

Diet 71

Exercise 72

Best Diet for Hypothyroidism: Foods to Eat, Foods to Avoid 74

Which nutrients are important? 79

Iodine 80

Selenium 81

Zinc 82

Which nutrients are harmful? 83

Goitrogens 83

Foods to avoid 85

Foods to eat 87

Sample meal plan 89

Tips for maintaining a healthy weight 93

Everything You Need to Know About Hypothyroidism

What is hypothyroidism?

Hypothyroidism occurs when your body doesn't produce enough thyroid hormones. The thyroid is a small, butterfly-shaped gland that sits at the front of your neck. It releases hormones to help your body regulate and use energy.

Your thyroid is responsible for providing energy to nearly every organ in your body. It controls functions like how your heart beats and how your digestive system works. Without the right amount of thyroid hormones, your body's natural functions begin to slow down.

Also called underactive thyroid, hypothyroidism affects women more frequently than men. It commonly affects people over the age of 60, but can begin at any age. It may be discovered through a routine blood test or after symptoms begin.

If you've recently been diagnosed with the condition, it's important to know that treatment is considered simple, safe, and effective. Most treatments rely on supplementing your low hormone levels with artificial varieties. These hormones will replace what your body isn't producing on its own and help return your body's functions to normal.

What are the signs and symptoms of hypothyroidism?

The signs and symptoms of hypothyroidism vary from person to person. The severity of the condition also affects which signs and symptoms appear and when. The symptoms are also sometimes difficult to identify.

Early symptoms can include weight gain and fatigue. Both become more common as you age, regardless of your thyroid's health. You may not realize that these changes are related to your thyroid until more symptoms appear.

For most people, symptoms of the condition progress gradually over many years. As the thyroid slows more and more, the symptoms may become more easily identified. Of course, many of these symptoms also become more common with age in general. If you suspect your symptoms are the result of a thyroid problem, it's important you talk with your doctor. They can order a blood test to determine if you have hypothyroidism.

The most common signs and symptoms of hypothyroidism include:

- fatigue
- depression
- constipation
- feeling cold
- dry skin
- weight gain
- muscle weakness
- decreased sweating
- slowed heart rate
- elevated blood cholesterol
- pain and stiffness in your joints
- dry, thinning hair
- impaired memory

- fertility difficulties or menstrual changes

- muscle stiffness, aches, and tenderness

- hoarseness

- puffy, sensitive face

What causes hypothyroidism?

Common causes of hypothyroidism include:

An autoimmune disease

Your immune system is designed to protect your body's cells against invading bacteria and viruses. When unknown bacteria or viruses enter your body, your immune system responds by sending out fighter cells to destroy the foreign cells.

Sometimes, your body confuses normal, healthy cells for invading cells. This is called an autoimmune response. If the autoimmune response isn't regulated or treated, your immune system can attack healthy tissues. This can cause serious medical issues, including conditions like hypothyroidism.

Hashimoto's disease is an autoimmune condition and the most common cause of an underactive thyroid. This disease attacks your thyroid gland and causes chronic thyroid inflammation. The inflammation can reduce thyroid function. It's common to find multiple family members with this same condition.

Treatment for hyperthyroidism

If your thyroid gland produces too much thyroid hormone, you have a condition known as hyperthyroidism. Treatment for this condition aims to reduce and normalize thyroid hormone production.

Sometimes, treatment can cause the levels of your thyroid hormone to remain low permanently. This often occurs after treatment with radioactive iodine.

Surgical removal of your thyroid

If your entire thyroid gland is removed due to thyroid problems, you'll develop hypothyroidism. Using thyroid medication for the rest of your life is the primary treatment.

If only a portion of the gland is removed, your thyroid may still be able to produce enough hormones on its own. Blood tests will help determine how much thyroid medication you'll need.

Radiation therapy

If you've been diagnosed with cancer of the head or neck, lymphoma, or leukemia, you may have undergone radiation therapy. Radiation used for the treatment of these conditions may slow or halt the production of thyroid hormone. This will almost always lead to hypothyroidism.

Medications

Several medicines may lower thyroid hormone production. These include ones used to treat psychological conditions, as well as cancer and heart disease. This can lead to hypothyroidism.

Diagnosing hypothyroidism

Two primary tools are used to determine if you have hypothyroidism:

Medical evaluation

Your doctor will complete a thorough physical exam and medical history. They'll check for physical signs of hypothyroidism, including:

- dry skin

- slowed reflexes

- swelling

- a slower heart rate

In addition, your doctor will ask you to report any symptoms you've been experiencing, such as fatigue, depression, constipation, or feeling constantly cold.

If you have a known family history of thyroid conditions, it's important you tell your doctor during this exam.

Blood tests

Blood tests are the only way to reliably confirm a diagnosis of hypothyroidism.

A thyroid-stimulating hormone (TSH) test measures how much TSH your pituitary gland is creating:

• If your thyroid isn't producing enough hormones, the pituitary gland will boost TSH to increase thyroid hormone production.

• If you have hypothyroidism, your TSH levels are high, as your body is trying to stimulate more thyroid hormone activity.

• If you have hyperthyroidism, your TSH levels are low, as your body is trying to stop excessive thyroid hormone production.

A thyroxine (T4) level test is also useful in diagnosing hypothyroidism. T4 is one of the hormones directly produced by your thyroid. Used together, T4 and TSH tests help evaluate thyroid function.

Typically, if you have a low level of T4 along with a high level of TSH, you have hypothyroidism. However, there is a spectrum of thyroid disease, and other thyroid function tests may be necessary to properly diagnose your condition.

Medications for hypothyroidism

Hypothyroidism is a lifelong condition. For many people, medication reduces or alleviates symptoms.

Hypothyroidism is best treated by using levothyroxine (Levothroid, Levoxyl). This synthetic version of the T4 hormone copies the action of the thyroid hormone your body would normally produce.

The medication is designed to return adequate levels of thyroid hormone to your blood. Once hormone levels are restored, symptoms of the condition are likely to disappear or at least become much more manageable.

Once you start treatment, it takes several weeks before you begin feeling relief. You'll require follow-up blood tests to monitor your progress. You and your doctor will work together to find a dose and a treatment plan that best addresses your symptoms. This can take some time.

In most cases, people with hypothyroidism must remain on this medication their entire lives. However, it's unlikely you'll continue to take the same dose. To make sure your medication is still working properly, your doctor should test your TSH levels yearly.

If blood levels indicate the medicine isn't working as well as it should, your doctor will adjust the dose until a balance is achieved.

Alternative treatment for hypothyroidism

Animal extracts that contain thyroid hormone are available. These extracts come from the thyroid glands of pigs. They contain both T4 and triiodothyronine (T3).

If you take levothyroxine, you're only receiving T4. But that's all you need because your body is capable of producing T3 from the synthetic T4.

These alterative animal extracts are often unreliable in dosing and haven't been shown in studies to be better than levothyroxine. For these reasons, they aren't routinely recommended.

Additionally, you can purchase glandular extracts in some health food stores. These products aren't monitored or regulated by the U.S. Food and Drug Administration. Because of this, their potency, legitimacy, and purity aren't guaranteed. Use these products at your own risk. But do tell your doctor if you decide to try these products so they can adjust your treatment accordingly.

Dietary recommendations for people with hypothyroidism

As a general rule, people with hypothyroidism don't have a specific diet they should follow. However, here are some recommendations to keep in mind:

Eat a balanced diet

Your thyroid needs adequate amounts of iodine in order to fully function. You don't need to take an iodine supplement in order for that to happen. A balanced diet of whole grains, beans, lean proteins, and colorful fruits and vegetables should provide enough iodine.

Monitor soy intake

Soy may hinder the absorption of thyroid hormones. If you drink or eat too many soy products, you may not be able to properly absorb your medication. This can be especially important in infants needing treatment for hypothyroidism who also drink soy formula.

Soy is found in:

- tofu

- vegan cheese and meat products

- soy milk

- soybeans

- soy sauce

You need steady doses of the medication to achieve even levels of thyroid hormone in your blood. Avoid eating or drinking soy-based foods for at least two hours before and after you take your medication.

Be smart with fiber

Like soy, fiber may interfere with hormone absorption. Too much dietary fiber may prevent your body from getting the hormones it needs. Fiber is important, so don't avoid it entirely. Instead, avoid taking your medicine within several hours of eating high-fiber foods.

Don't take thyroid medicine with other supplements

If you take supplements or medications in addition to thyroid medicine, try to take these medicines at different times. Other medications can interfere with absorption, so it's best to take your thyroid medicine on an empty stomach and without other medicines or foods.

Living with hypothyroidism: Things to consider

Even if you're undergoing treatment, you may deal with long-lasting issues or complications because of the condition. There are ways to lessen the effect of hypothyroidism on your quality of life:

Develop fatigue coping strategies

Despite taking medication, you may still experience fatigue from time to time. It's important you get quality sleep each night, eat a diet rich in fruits and vegetables, and consider the use of stress-relieving mechanisms, like meditation and yoga, to help you combat low energy levels.

Talk it out

Having a chronic medical condition can be difficult, especially if it's accompanied by other health concerns. Find people you can openly express your feelings and experiences to. This can be a therapist, close friend, or family member, or a support group of other people living with this condition.

Many hospitals sponsor meetings for people with conditions like hypothyroidism. Ask for a recommendation from your hospital's education office, and attend a meeting. You may be able to connect with people who understand exactly what you're experiencing and can offer a guiding hand.

Monitor for other health conditions

There is a link between other autoimmune diseases and hypothyroidism.

Hypothyroidism often goes along with other conditions like:

- celiac disease

- diabetes

- rheumatoid arthritis

- lupus

- adrenal gland disorders

- pituitary problems

- obstructive sleep apnea

Hypothyroidism and depression

When levels of thyroid hormones are low, your body's natural functions slow down and lag. This creates a variety of symptoms, including fatigue, weight gain, even depression.

Some people with hypothyroidism may only experience mood difficulties. This can make diagnosing hypothyroidism difficult. Instead of only treating the brain, doctors should also consider testing for and treating an underactive thyroid.

Depression and hypothyroidism share several symptoms. These include:

- difficulty concentrating
- weight gain
- fatigue

- depressed mood

- reduced desire and satisfaction

- sleep difficulties

The two conditions also have symptoms that may distinguish them from one another. For hypothyroidism, problems such as dry skin, constipation, high cholesterol, and hair loss are common. For depression alone, these conditions wouldn't be expected.

Depression is often a diagnosis made based on symptoms and medical history. Low thyroid function is diagnosed with a physical exam and blood tests. To see if there's a link between your depression and your thyroid function, your doctor can order these tests for a definitive diagnosis.

If your depression is caused only by hypothyroidism, correcting the hypothyroidism should treat the depression. If it doesn't, your doctor may prescribe medications for both conditions. They'll slowly adjust your doses until your depression and hypothyroidism come under control.

Hypothyroidism and anxiety

While hypothyroidism has long been associated with depression, a recent study indicates it may be associated with anxiety, too. Researchers recently evaluated 100 patients between the ages of 18 and 45 with a known history of hypothyroidism. Using an anxiety questionnaire, they found that nearly 60 percent of people with hypothyroidism met the criteria for some form of anxiety.

The research to date has consisted of small studies. Larger and more focused studies on anxiety may help determine if a true connection exists between hypothyroidism and anxiety. It's important for you and your doctor to discuss all your symptoms when being evaluated for thyroid conditions.

Hypothyroidism and pregnancy

Hypothyroidism affects your entire body. Your thyroid is responsible for many of your body's daily functions, including metabolism, heartbeat, and temperature control. When your body doesn't produce enough thyroid hormone, all of these functions can slow.

Women who have hypothyroidism and wish to become pregnant face a particular set of challenges. Low thyroid function or uncontrolled hypothyroidism during pregnancy can cause:

- anemia
- miscarriage
- preeclampsia
- stillbirth
- low birth weight
- brain development problems
- birth defects

Women with thyroid problems can and very often do have healthy pregnancies. If you have hypothyroidism and are pregnant, it's important to keep the following in mind during the time you're expecting:

Stay current on medicine

Continue to take your medication as prescribed. It's common to have frequent testing so your doctor can make any necessary adjustments to your thyroid medication as your pregnancy progresses.

Talk to your doctor about testing

Women can develop hypothyroidism while they're pregnant. This occurs in three to five out of every 1,000 pregnancies. Some doctors routinely check thyroid levels during pregnancy to monitor for low thyroid hormone levels. If the levels are lower than they should be, your doctor may suggest treatment.

Some women who never had thyroid problems before they were pregnant may develop them after having a baby. This is called postpartum thyroiditis. In about 80 percent of women, the condition resolves after a year, and medication is no longer required. Approximately 20 percent of women who have this diagnosis will go on to require long-term therapy.

Eat well

Your body needs more nutrients, vitamins, and minerals while you're pregnant. Eating a well-balanced diet and taking multivitamins while you're pregnant can help maintain a healthy pregnancy.

Hypothyroidism and weight loss

Your thyroid gland creates hormones that are responsible for a large number of bodily functions. These functions include using energy, controlling body temperature, keeping organs functioning, and regulating metabolism.

When thyroid hormone levels are low, research shows that people are more likely to gain weight. That's likely because their body doesn't burn energy as efficiently as a body with a healthier thyroid. The amount of weight gain isn't very high, however. Most people will gain somewhere between 5 and 10 pounds.

Once you're treated for this condition, you may lose any weight that you've gained. If treatment doesn't help eliminate the extra weight, you should be able to lose weight with a change in diet and an increase in exercise. That's because once your thyroid levels are restored, your ability to manage your weight returns to normal.

Hypothyroidism and weight gain

When your thyroid doesn't function as well as it should, many of your body's functions slow down. This includes the rate at which you use energy, or metabolic rate.

If your thyroid gland doesn't function properly, your resting or basal metabolic rate may be low. For that reason, an underactive thyroid is commonly associated with weight gain. The more severe the condition is, the greater your weight gain is likely to be.

Properly treating the condition can help you lose any weight you gained while your thyroid levels were uncontrolled. However, it's important to know that's not always the case. Symptoms of underactive thyroid, including weight gain, develop over a long period of time.

It's not uncommon for people with low thyroid hormone to lose no weight once they find treatment for the condition. That doesn't mean the condition isn't being properly treated. Instead, the weight gain may be the result of lifestyle rather than low hormone levels.

If you've been diagnosed with hypothyroidism and are treating the condition but don't see a change in your weight, you can still lose weight. Work with your doctor, registered dietitian, or personal trainer to develop a focused healthy-eating plan and exercise strategy that can help you lose weight.

Facts and statistics about hypothyroidism

Hypothyroidism is a fairly common condition. About 4.6 percent of Americans ages 12 and over have hypothyroidism. That's about 10 million people in the United States living with the condition.

The disease gets more common with age. People over age 60 experience it more frequently.

Women are more likely to have an underactive thyroid. In fact, 1 in 5 women will develop hypothyroidism by age 60.

One of the most common causes of an underactive thyroid gland is Hashimoto's disease. It affects middle-aged women most commonly, but it can occur in men and children. This condition also runs in families. If a family member has been diagnosed with this disease, your risk for having it is higher.

It's important to pay attention to changes your body goes through during your life span. If you notice a significant difference in how you feel or how your body is responding, talk to your doctor to see if a thyroid problem may be affecting you.

10 Signs and Symptoms of Hypothyroidism

Thyroid disorders are common. In fact, about 12% of people will experience abnormal thyroid function at some point during their lives.

Women are eight times more likely to develop a thyroid disorder than men. Also, thyroid problems increase with age and may affect adults differently than children.

At the most basic level, thyroid hormone is responsible for coordinating energy, growth and metabolism in your body.

Problems can occur when this hormone's levels are too high or low.

Hypothyroidism, or low levels of thyroid hormone, slows your metabolism and decreases growth or repair of many parts of the body.

The thyroid is a small, butterfly-shaped gland that drapes across the front of your windpipe.

If you place your fingers on the sides of your Adam's apple and swallow, you'll feel your thyroid gland sliding under your fingers.

It releases thyroid hormone, which controls the growth and metabolism of essentially every part of your body.

The pituitary, a tiny gland in the middle of your head, monitors your physiology and releases thyroid-stimulating hormone (TSH). TSH is the signal to the thyroid gland to release thyroid hormone (1Trusted Source).

Sometimes TSH levels increase, but the thyroid gland can't release more thyroid hormone in response. This is known as primary hypothyroidism, as the problem begins at the level of the thyroid gland.

Other times, TSH levels decrease, and the thyroid never receives the signal to increase thyroid hormone levels. This is called secondary hypothyroidism.

Hypothyroidism, or "low thyroid," can cause a variety of signs and symptoms. This article will help you recognize and understand these effects.

Here are 10 common signs and symptoms of hypothyroidism.

1. Feeling Tired

One of the most common symptoms of hypothyroidism is feeling worn out. Thyroid hormone controls energy balance and can influence whether you feel ready to go or ready to nap.

As an extreme example, animals that hibernate experience low thyroid levels leading up to their long sleep.

Thyroid hormone receives signals from the brain and coordinates cells to change their functions, depending on what else is going on in your body.

Those with high levels of thyroid hormone feel nervous and jittery. In contrast, people with low thyroid feel exhausted and sluggish.

In one study, 138 adults with hypothyroidism experienced physical exhaustion and reduced activity. They also reported low motivation and feeling mentally tired.

Low-thyroid individuals feel unrested, even though they may be sleeping more.

In another study, 50% of people with hypothyroidism felt constantly tired, while 42% of people with low thyroid hormone said they slept more than they used to.

Feeling sleepier than usual without a good explanation could be a sign of hypothyroidism.

SUMMARY:

Thyroid hormone is like a gas pedal for energy and metabolism. Low thyroid hormone levels leave you feeling drained.

2. Gaining Weight

Unexpected weight gain is another common symptom of hypothyroidism.

Not only are low-thyroid individuals moving less — they're also signaling their livers, muscles and fat tissue to hold on to calories.

When thyroid levels are low, metabolism switches modes. Instead of burning calories for growth and activity, the amount of energy you use at rest, or your basal metabolic rate, decreases. As a result, your body tends to store more calories from the diet as fat.

Because of this, low thyroid hormone levels can cause weight gain, even if the number of calories eaten remains constant.

In fact, in one study, people with newly diagnosed hypothyroidism gained an average of 15–30 pounds (7–14 kg) in the year since their diagnoses.

If you've been experiencing weight gain, first consider whether other changes in your lifestyle might explain it.

If you seem to be gaining weight in spite of a good diet and exercise plan, bring it up with your doctor. It might be a clue that something else is going on.

SUMMARY:

Hypothyroidism signals the body to eat more, store calories and burn fewer calories. This combination leads to weight gain.

3. Feeling Cold

Heat is a byproduct of burning calories.

For example, consider how hot you get when you workout. This is because you are burning calories.

Even when you're sitting, you're burning a small amount of calories. However, in cases of hypothyroidism, your basal metabolic rate decreases, reducing the amount of heat you generate.

In addition, thyroid hormone turns up the thermostat on brown fat, which is a specialized type of fat that generates heat. Brown fat is important in maintaining body heat in cold climates, but hypothyroidism prevents it from doing its job.

That's why low levels of thyroid hormone cause you to feel colder than others around you. About 40% of low-thyroid individuals feel more sensitive to cold than usual.

If you've always wanted the room warmer than the people you live and work with, this may just be the way you are built.

But if you've noticed yourself feeling colder than normal lately, it could be a sign of hypothyroidism.

SUMMARY:

Low thyroid hormone slows down your body's normal heat production, leaving you cold.

4. Weakness and Aches in Muscles and Joints

Low thyroid hormone flips the metabolic switch toward catabolism, which is when the body breaks down body tissues like muscle for energy.

During catabolism, muscle strength decreases, potentially leading to feelings of weakness. The process of breaking down muscle tissue can also lead to aching.

Everyone feels weak once in a while. However, people with hypothyroidism are twice as likely to feel more weak than usual, compared to healthy people.

Additionally, 34% of low-thyroid individuals get muscle cramps in the absence of recent activity.

One study in 35 individuals with hypothyroidism showed that replacing low levels of thyroid hormone with a synthetic thyroid hormone called levothyroxine improved muscle strength and decreased aches and pains, compared to no treatment.

Another study showed a 25% improvement in the sense of physical well-being among patients receiving thyroid replacement.

Weakness and aches are normal following strenuous activity. However, new, and especially increasing, weakness or aching is a good reason to make an appointment with your physician.

SUMMARY:

Low levels of thyroid hormone slow down your metabolism and can cause painful muscle breakdown.

5. Hair Loss

Like most cells, hair follicles are regulated by thyroid hormone.

Because hair follicles have stem cells that have a short lifespan and rapid turnover, they are more sensitive to low thyroid levels than other tissues (14Trusted Source).

Low thyroid hormone causes hair follicles to stop regenerating, resulting in hair loss. This will typically improve when the thyroid issue is treated.

In one study, about 25–30% of patients seeing a specialist for hair loss were found to have low thyroid hormone. This increased to 40% in individuals over 40 (15Trusted Source).

Furthermore, another study showed that hypothyroidism may cause coarsening of the hair in up to 10% of individuals with low thyroid hormone (6Trusted Source).

Consider hypothyroidism if you experience unexpected changes in the rate or pattern of your hair loss, particularly if your hair becomes patchy or coarser.

Other hormone problems can also cause unexpected hair loss. Your doctor can help you sort out whether your hair loss is anything to worry about.

SUMMARY: Low thyroid hormone affects rapidly growing cells like hair follicles. This can cause hair loss and coarsening of the hair.

6. Itchy and Dry Skin

Like hair follicles, skin cells are characterized by rapid turnover. Therefore, they are also sensitive to losing growth signals from the thyroid hormone.

When the normal cycle of skin renewal is broken, skin may take longer to regrow.

This means the outer layer of skin has been around longer, accumulating damage. It also means that dead skin may take longer to shed, leading to flaky, dry skin.

One study showed 74% of low-thyroid individuals reported dry skin. However, 50% of patients with normal thyroid levels also reported dry skin from other causes, making it hard to know if thyroid problems were the cause.

Additionally, the study showed that 50% of people with hypothyroidism reported that their skin had gotten worse over the past year.

Changes in skin that cannot be blamed on allergies like hay fever or new products can be a more practical sign of thyroid problems.

Finally, hypothyroidism is sometimes caused by autoimmune disease. This can affect the skin, causing swelling and redness known as myxedema. Myxedema is more specific to thyroid problems than other causes of dry skin (16Trusted Source).

SUMMARY:Hypothyroidism commonly causes dry skin. However, most people with dry skin do not have hypothyroidism. Myxedema is a red, swollen rash that is characteristic of thyroid problems.

7. Feeling Down or Depressed

Hypothyroidism is linked to depression. The reasons for this are unclear, but it might be a mental symptom of an overall decrease in energy and health (17Trusted Source).

64% of women and 57% of men with hypothyroidism report feelings of depression. About the same percentage of men and women also experience anxiety (18).

In one study, thyroid hormone replacement improved depression in patients with mild hypothyroidism, compared to a placebo (19).

Another study of young women with mild hypothyroidism showed increased feelings of depression, which were also connected to decreased satisfaction with their sex lives (18).

Furthermore, postpartum hormone fluctuations are a common cause of hypothyroidism, potentially contributing to postpartum depression.

Feeling depressed is a good reason to talk to a physician or therapist. They may be able to help you cope, regardless of whether the depression is caused by thyroid problems or something else.

SUMMARY: Hypothyroidism can cause depression and anxiety. These conditions are shown to improve with thyroid hormone replacement.

8. Trouble Concentrating or Remembering

Many patients with hypothyroidism complain of mental "fogginess" and trouble concentrating. The way this mental fogginess presents itself varies by person.

In one study, 22% of low-thyroid individuals described increased difficulty doing everyday math, 36% described thinking more slowly than usual and 39% reported having a poorer memory.

In another study of 14 men and women with untreated hypothyroidism, the participants showed difficulty remembering verbal cues (4).

The causes for this are not yet fully understood, but difficulties in memory improve with treatment of low thyroid hormone.

Difficulties in memory or concentration can happen to everyone, but if they are sudden or severe, they could be a signal of hypothyroidism.

SUMMARY:

Hypothyroidism can cause mental fogginess and difficulty concentrating. It may also impair certain kinds of memory.

9. Constipation

Low thyroid levels put the brakes on your colon.

According to one study, constipation affects 17% of people with low thyroid hormone, compared to 10% of people with normal thyroid levels (6Trusted Source).

In this study, 20% of people with hypothyroidism said their constipation was getting worse, compared to only 6% of normal-thyroid individuals (6Trusted Source).

While constipation is a common complaint in patients with hypothyroidism, it's uncommon for constipation to be the only or most severe symptom (24Trusted Source).

If you experience constipation but otherwise feel fine, try these natural laxatives before worrying about your thyroid.

If they don't work, your constipation worsens, you go several days without passing a stool or you begin having stomach pain or vomiting, seek medical advice.

SUMMARY:

Most people with constipation don't have hypothyroidism. However, if constipation is accompanied by other signs of hypothyroidism, your thyroid may be the cause.

10. Heavy or Irregular Periods

Both irregular and heavy menstrual bleeding are linked to hypothyroidism.

One study showed that about 40% of women with low thyroid hormone experienced increasing menstrual irregularity or heavy bleeding in the last year, compared to 26% of women with normal thyroid levels (6Trusted Source).

In another study, 30% of women with hypothyroidism had irregular and heavy periods. These women had been diagnosed with hypothyroidism after other symptoms had caused them to get tested (25Trusted Source).

Thyroid hormone interacts with other hormones that control the menstrual cycle, and abnormal levels of it can disrupt their signals. Also, thyroid hormone directly affects the ovaries and uterus.

There are several problems besides hypothyroidism that can cause heavy or irregular periods. If you have irregular or heavy periods that disrupt your lifestyle, consider talking with a gynecologist before worrying about your thyroid.

SUMMARY:

Heavy periods or irregular cycles that are worse than usual could be caused by a medical condition, including hypothyroidism. It's best to talk to a gynecologist about them.

The Bottom Line

Hypothyroidism, or low thyroid, is a common disorder.

It can cause a variety of symptoms, such as fatigue, weight gain and feeling cold. It can also result in problems with your hair, skin, muscles, memory or mood.

Importantly, none of these problems are unique to hypothyroidism.

Yet if you are having several of these symptoms or they are new, worsening or severe, see your doctor to decide if you need to be tested for hypothyroidism.

Fortunately, hypothyroidism is generally treatable with inexpensive medications.

If your thyroid hormone levels are low, a simple treatment could greatly improve your quality of life.

Your Hypothyroidism Diet Plan: Eat This, Not That

Hypothyroidism treatment typically starts with taking replacement thyroid hormone, but it doesn't end there. You also need to watch what you eat. Sticking to a healthy diet can prevent the weight gain that often comes with having an underactive thyroid. Avoiding certain foods can help your replacement thyroid hormone work as well as it should.

Here's a look at some foods to add to or remove from your hypothyroidism diet plan.

What to eat

There is no specific hypothyroidism diet. Eating a low-fat diet with a good balance of fruits, vegetables, lean protein (fish, poultry, lean meat), dairy, and whole grains is a good strategy for everyone to follow.

You also want to balance your calorie intake. Portion control is essential to preventing weight gain. Hypothyroidism slows your metabolism, and you can put on a few pounds unless you burn off more calories than you take in each day. Talk to your doctor or work with a dietitian to figure out how many calories you should eat each day, and what foods will help you feel your best.

What to limit or avoid

Hypothyroidism does come with a few dietary restrictions. First, you'll want to avoid high-fat, processed, and sugary foods that can contribute to weight gain. Also limit salt to no more than 2,300 milligrams daily. Too much salt can raise your blood pressure, which is already a risk when your thyroid is underactive.

Here are a few foods to limit or avoid, because they can affect how well your thyroid gland or your thyroid replacement hormone works.

Iodine

Your thyroid needs iodine to make its hormones. Though your body doesn't make this element, it's found in a variety of foods, including iodized table salt, cheese, fish, and ice cream. If you eat a normal diet, you shouldn't become deficient in iodine.

Yet you don't want to eat too much, either. Taking iodine supplements or eating too many foods that contain iron can lead to hyperthyroidism — an overactive thyroid gland. Also avoid supplements that contain kelp, a type of seaweed that's high in iodine.

Soy

Soy-based foods like tofu and soybean flour are high in protein, low in fat, and rich in nutrients. However, they also contain the female hormone estrogen, which could interfere with your body's absorption of synthetic thyroid hormone.

Though you don't need to stop eating soy entirely, your doctor might recommend that you limit the amount you eat, or adjust when you eat it. Wait at least four hours after taking your hypothyroidism medicine before consuming any soy foods.

Fiber

Too much fiber can interfere with the absorption of your thyroid hormone medicine. Current dietary recommendations call for 25 grams of fiber daily for women, and 38 grams for men. Ask your doctor or dietitian how much you should eat each day.

Don't stop eating fiber entirely — it's found in healthy foods like fruits, vegetables, beans, and whole grain breads and cereals. Just don't overdo it. And wait a few hours after taking your thyroid medicine before you eat high-fiber foods.

Cruciferous vegetables

Brussels sprouts, broccoli, and cabbage are part of the cruciferous family of vegetables. These vegetables are high in fiber and vitamins, and they may help protect against cancer and other diseases. Cruciferous vegetables have been linked to hypothyroidism — but only when eaten in very large amounts. If you make them just one part of a wide variety of vegetables in your diet, they shouldn't be a problem.

Alcohol

Alcohol doesn't interact with levothyroxine, but if you drink too much, it can damage your liver. Because your liver breaks down drugs like thyroid hormone to remove them from your body, alcohol-induced liver damage could lead to too much levothyroxine in your system. Check with your doctor to see whether it's safe for you to have alcohol, and how much you can drink.

Gluten

Gluten — the protein found in grains like wheat, rye, and barley — doesn't directly affect thyroid function. Yet some people with autoimmune hypothyroidism also have celiac disease, a condition in which their immune system mistakenly attacks their small intestine after they eat gluten.

If you have symptoms like abdominal bloating, stomachache, diarrhea, and vomiting after you eat foods containing gluten, see your doctor for a celiac blood test. Eliminating gluten from your diet should relieve these symptoms.

Iron and calcium

Both of these minerals can interfere with the absorption of your thyroid hormone medicine. While foods containing iron and calcium are safe to eat, avoid them in supplement form.

Planning your diet

When you have a chronic condition like hypothyroidism, don't try to navigate your diet alone. Start with a visit to your doctor, who can help you identify which foods might cause interactions or other problems with your thyroid medicine. Then work with a dietitian, who can help you develop a diet that's both healthy and thyroid friendly.

Your Treatment Options for Hypothyroidism

Hypothyroidism is a condition where the thyroid gland doesn't produce or make enough of two thyroid hormones: triiodothyronine (T3) and thyroxine (T4). The thyroid gland is a small organ at the base of the throat that's responsible for regulating your metabolism. The pituitary gland secretes a thyroid-stimulating hormone (TSH) that triggers the thyroid to make and release T3 and T4.

Primary hypothyroidism occurs when the thyroid doesn't make enough T3 and T4 despite being instructed to do so by the pituitary gland. Secondary hypothyroidism occurs when there's too little TSH stimulating the thyroid gland. Common symptoms of the condition include fatigue, body pain, palpitations, and menstrual irregularity. Although there may be no cure for hypothyroidism, there are ways to control it.

Medications and Supplements

Using synthetic versions of the thyroid hormones is one of the most commonly used treatments for hypothyroidism. Liothyronine (Cytomel, Tertroxin) is a synthetic version of T3 and levothyroxine (Synthroid, Levothroid, Levoxyl) is a substitute for T4.

If your hypothyroidism is caused by an iodine deficiency, your doctor may recommend an iodine supplement. Additionally, magnesium and selenium supplements may help improve your condition. As always, ask your doctor before taking any supplements.

Diet

Although many foods can improve thyroid function, changes to your diet are unlikely to replace the need for prescription medication.

Nuts and seeds rich in magnesium and selenium, including Brazil nuts and sunflower seeds, can be beneficial to your thyroid health.

Dietary supplements, like iron and calcium pills, and eating a high-fiber diet can reduce the absorption of certain thyroid medicines. In general, avoid eating soy and soy-based foods, kale, broccoli, cauliflower, and cabbage as these foods can inhibit thyroid function, especially when eaten in raw form.

Exercise

Hypothyroidism can trigger muscle and joint pain and can leave you feeling fatigued and depressed. A regular exercise routine can reduce many of these symptoms.

Unless your doctor advises you against certain activities, no exercises are off-limits. Still, the following activities may be especially helpful for hypothyroidism.

Low-impact workouts: One of the common symptoms of hypothyroidism is muscle and joint pain. Biking, swimming, yoga, Pilates, or walking at a brisk pace are just some low-impact activities that you can incorporate into your everyday routine.

Strength training: Building muscle mass, either by lifting weights or with exercises such as push-ups and pull-ups, can reduce any feelings of sluggishness or lethargy.

Having a higher muscle mass increases your resting metabolic rate, which can help counter any weight gain and pains caused by hypothyroidism.

Cardiovascular training: Hypothyroidism has been correlated with a higher risk of cardiac arrhythmias, or an irregular heartbeat. Improving your cardiovascular health with regular exercise can help protect your heart.

Through medications, diet, and exercise, you can improve your thyroid health and manage your hypothyroidism.

Best Diet for Hypothyroidism: Foods to Eat, Foods to Avoid

Hypothyroidism is a condition in which the body doesn't make enough thyroid hormones.

Thyroid hormones help control growth, cell repair, and metabolism. As a result, people with hypothyroidism may experience tiredness, hair loss, weight gain, feeling cold, and feeling down, among many other symptoms.

Hypothyroidism affects 1–2% of people worldwide and is ten times more likely to affect women than men.

Foods alone won't cure hypothyroidism. However, a combination of the right nutrients and medication can help restore thyroid function and minimize your symptoms.

This article outlines the best diet for hypothyroidism, including which foods to eat and which to avoid — all based on research.

The thyroid gland is a small, butterfly-shaped gland that sits near the base of your neck.

It makes and stores thyroid hormones that affect nearly every cell in your body.

When the thyroid gland receives a signal called thyroid-stimulating hormone (TSH), it releases thyroid hormones into the bloodstream. This signal is sent from the pituitary gland, a small gland found at the base of your brain, when thyroid hormone levels are low (4Trusted Source).

Occasionally, the thyroid gland doesn't release thyroid hormones, even when there is plenty of TSH. This is called primary hypothyroidism and the most common type of hypothyroidism.

Approximately 90% of primary hypothyroidism is caused by Hashimoto's thyroiditis, an autoimmune disease in which your immune system mistakenly attacks your thyroid gland.

Other causes of primary hypothyroidism are iodine deficiency, a genetic disorder, taking certain medications, and surgery that removes part of the thyroid.

Other times, the thyroid gland does not receive enough TSH. This happens when the pituitary gland is not working properly and is called secondary hypothyroidism.

Thyroid hormones are very important. They help control growth, cell repair, and metabolism — the process by which your body converts what you eat into energy.

Your metabolism affects your body temperature and at what rate you burn calories. That's why people with hypothyroidism often feel cold and fatigued and may gain weight easily.

You can learn more about the signs and symptoms of hypothyroidism here.

SUMMARY

Hypothyroidism is a condition in which the thyroid gland does not make enough thyroid hormone. As the thyroid hormone is important for growth, repair, and metabolism, people with hypothyroidism may often feel cold and fatigued and may gain weight easily.

How does hypothyroidism affect your metabolism?

The thyroid hormone helps control the speed of your metabolism. The faster your metabolism, the more calories your body burns at rest.

People with hypothyroidism make less thyroid hormone. This means they have a slower metabolism and burn fewer calories at rest.

Having a slow metabolism comes with several health risks. It may leave you tired, increase your blood cholesterol levels, and make it harder for you to lose weight.

If you find it difficult to maintain your weight with hypothyroidism, try doing moderate or high intensity cardio. This includes exercises like fast-paced walking, running, hiking, and rowing.

Research shows that moderate to high intensity aerobic exercise may help boost your thyroid hormone levels. In turn, this may help speed up your metabolism.

People with hypothyroidism might also benefit from increasing their protein intake. Research shows that higher protein diets help increase the rate of your metabolism.

SUMMARY

People with hypothyroidism usually have a slower metabolism. Research shows that aerobic exercise can help boost your thyroid hormone levels. Additionally, eating more protein may help boost your metabolism.

Which nutrients are important?

Several nutrients are important for optimal thyroid health.

Iodine

Iodine is an essential mineral that's needed to make thyroid hormones. Thus, people with iodine deficiency might be at risk of hypothyroidism (11Trusted Source).

Iodine deficiency is very common and affects nearly one-third of the world's population. However, it's less common in people from developed countries like the United States, where iodized salt and iodine-rich seafood is widely available.

If you have an iodine deficiency, consider adding iodized table salt to your meals or eating more iodine-rich foods like seaweed, fish, dairy, and eggs.

Iodine supplements are unnecessary, as you can get plenty of iodine from your diet. Some studies have also shown that getting too much of this mineral may damage the thyroid gland.

Selenium

Selenium helps "activate" thyroid hormones so they can be used by the body (14Trusted Source).

This essential mineral also has antioxidant benefits, which means it may protect the thyroid gland from damage by molecules called free radicals.

Adding selenium-rich foods to your diet is a great way to boost your selenium levels. This includes Brazil nuts, tuna, sardines, eggs, and legumes.

However, avoid taking a selenium supplement unless advised by your healthcare provider. Supplements provide large doses, and selenium may be toxic in large amounts.

Zinc

Like selenium, zinc helps the body "activate" thyroid hormones.

Studies also show that zinc may help the body regulate TSH, the hormone that tells the thyroid gland to release thyroid hormones.

Zinc deficiencies are rare in developed countries, as zinc is abundant in the food supply.

Nonetheless, if you have hypothyroidism, you should aim to eat more zinc-rich foods like oysters and other shellfish, beef, and chicken.

SUMMARY

Research shows that iodine, selenium, and zinc are especially beneficial for those with hypothyroidism. However, it's best to avoid iodine and selenium supplements unless your healthcare provider advises you to take them.

Which nutrients are harmful?

Several nutrients may harm the health of those with hypothyroidism.

Goitrogens

Goitrogens are compounds that may interfere with the normal function of the thyroid gland.

They get their name from the term goiter, which is an enlarged thyroid gland that may occur with hypothyroidism.

Surprisingly, many common foods contain goitrogens, including:

- soy foods: tofu, tempeh, edamame, etc.

- certain vegetables: cabbage, broccoli, kale, cauliflower, spinach, etc.

- fruits and starchy plants: sweet potatoes, cassava, peaches, strawberries, etc.

- nuts and seeds: millet, pine nuts, peanuts, etc.

In theory, people with hypothyroidism should avoid goitrogens. However, this only seems to be an issue for people who have an iodine deficiency or eat large amounts of goitrogens.

Also, cooking foods with goitrogens may inactivate these compounds.

One exception to the above foods is pearl millet. Some studies have found that pearl millet might interfere with thyroid function, even if you don't have an iodine deficiency.

SUMMARY

Dietary substances that may affect thyroid function include goitrogens.

Foods to avoid

Fortunately, you don't have to avoid many foods if you have hypothyroidism.

However, foods that contain goitrogens should be eaten in moderation and ideally cooked.

You should also avoid eating highly processed foods, as they usually contain a lot of calories. This can be a problem if you have hypothyroidism, as you may gain weight easily.

Here is a list of foods and supplements you should avoid:

- millet: all varieties

- highly processed foods: hot dogs, cakes, cookies, etc.

- supplements: Adequate intakes of selenium and iodine are essential for thyroid health, but getting too much of either may cause harm. Only supplement with selenium and iodine if your healthcare provider has instructed you to do so.

Here is a list of foods you can eat in moderation. These foods contain goitrogens or are known irritants if consumed in large amounts.

- soy-based foods: tofu, tempeh, edamame beans, soy milk, etc.

- cruciferous vegetables: broccoli, kale, spinach, cabbage, etc.

- certain fruits: peaches, pears, and strawberries

- beverages: coffee, green tea, and alcohol — these beverages may irritate your thyroid gland

SUMMARY

People with hypothyroidism should avoid millet, processed foods, and supplements like selenium and zinc (unless a healthcare provider has advised you to take them). Foods that contain goitrogens are fine in moderate amounts unless they cause discomfort.

Foods to eat

There are plenty of food options for people with hypothyroidism, including:

- eggs: whole eggs are best, as much of their iodine and selenium are found in the yolk, while the whites are full of protein

- meat: all meats, including lamb, beef, chicken, etc.

- fish: all seafood, including salmon, tuna, halibut, shrimp, etc.

- vegetables: all vegetables — cruciferous vegetables are fine to eat in moderate amounts, especially when cooked

- fruits: all other fruits, including berries, bananas, oranges, tomatoes, etc.

- gluten-free grains and seeds: rice, buckwheat, quinoa, chia seeds, and flax seeds

- dairy: all dairy products, including milk, cheese, yogurt, etc.

- beverages: water and other non-caffeinated beverages

People with hypothyroidism should eat a diet based around vegetables, fruits, and lean meats. They are low in calories and very filling, which may help prevent weight gain.

SUMMARY

People with hypothyroidism have plenty of healthy food options, including eggs, meat, fish, most fruits and vegetables, gluten-free grains and seeds, all dairy products, and non-caffeinated beverages.

Sample meal plan

Here is a 7-day meal plan for those with hypothyroidism.

It provides a healthy amount of protein, has a low to moderate amount of carbs, and should help you maintain a healthy weight.

Make sure you take your thyroid medication at least 1–2 hours before your first meal, or as your healthcare provider has advised. Nutrients like fiber, calcium, and iron may stop your body from absorbing thyroid medication properly (30Trusted Source).

Monday

- breakfast: toast with eggs

- lunch: chicken salad with 2–3 Brazil nuts

- dinner: stir-fried chicken and vegetables served with rice

Tuesday

- breakfast: oatmeal with 1/4 cup (31 grams) of berries

- lunch: grilled salmon salad

- dinner: fish baked with lemon, thyme, and black pepper served with steamed vegetables

Wednesday

- breakfast: toast with eggs

- lunch: leftovers from dinner

- dinner: shrimp skewers served with a quinoa salad

Thursday

- breakfast: overnight chia pudding — 2 tbsp (28 grams) of chia seeds, 1 cup (240 ml) of Greek yogurt, 1/2 tsp of vanilla extract, and sliced fruits of your choice. Let sit in a bowl or mason jar overnight
- lunch: leftovers from dinner
- dinner: roast lamb served with steamed vegetables

Friday

- breakfast: banana-berry smoothie
- lunch: chicken salad sandwich
- dinner: pork fajitas — sliced lean pork, bell peppers, and salsa — served in corn tortillas

Saturday

- breakfast: egg, mushroom, and zucchini frittata
- lunch: tuna and boiled egg salad
- dinner: homemade Mediterranean pizza topped with tomato paste, olives, and feta cheese

Sunday

- breakfast: omelet with various vegetables
- lunch: quinoa salad with green vegetables and nuts
- dinner: grilled steak with a side salad

SUMMARY

This sample week-long meal plan is suitable for those with hypothyroidism. It provides plenty of options for a delicious and healthy menu.

Tips for maintaining a healthy weight

It's very easy to gain weight with hypothyroidism due to a slow metabolism.

Here are a few tips to help you maintain a healthy weight.

• Get plenty of rest. Aim to get 7–8 hours of sleep every night. Sleeping less than this is linked to fat gain, especially around the belly area.

• Practice mindful eating. Mindful eating, which involves paying attention to what you're eating, why you're eating, and how fast you're eating can help you develop a better relationship with food. Studies also show that it can help you lose weight.

• Try yoga or meditation. Yoga and meditation can help you de-stress and improve your overall health. Research also shows that they help you maintain a healthy weight (43Trusted Source).

- Try a low to moderate carb diet. Eating a low to moderate amount of carbs is very effective for maintaining a healthy weight. However, avoid trying a ketogenic diet, as eating too few carbs may lower your thyroid hormone levels.

SUMMARY

While it's easy to gain weight when you have hypothyroidism, plenty of strategies can help you maintain a healthy weight. For example, you can try getting plenty of rest, eating a good amount of protein, and practicing mindful eating.

The bottom line

Hypothyroidism, or an underactive thyroid, is a health problem that affects 1–2% of people worldwide.

It can cause symptoms like tiredness, weight gain, and feeling cold, among many others.

Fortunately, eating the right nutrients and taking medications may help reduce your symptoms and improve your thyroid function.

Nutrients that are great for your thyroid are iodine, selenium, and zinc.

Following a thyroid-friendly diet can minimize your symptoms and help you maintain a healthy weight. It encourages eating whole, unprocessed foods and lean protein.

Printed in Great Britain
by Amazon